17 95

Everything You Need to Know About

GOING
TO THE
GYNECOLOGIST

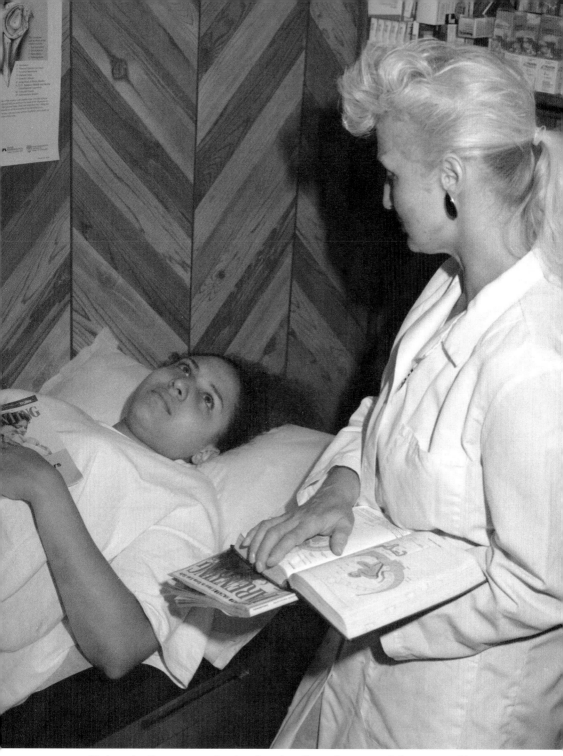

Going to the gynecologist for the first time won't be scary if you know the facts.

Everything You Need to Know About

GOING TO THE GYNECOLOGIST

Shifra N. Diamond

THE ROSEN PUBLISHING GROUP, INC.
NEW YORK

Research assistance for this book was provided by Mary Lewis, RN, CNM, MS, Director of Nurse-Midwifery Services at Hutzel Hospital, the Detroit Medical Center, and by Adelaide Nardone, MD, FACOG, gynecologist at the Women's Medical Associates of Westchester in Mount Kisco, NY. Dr. Nardone is also a consultant to the Vagisil Women's Health Center; she answers teens' questions about gynecology at http://www.vagisil.com. The author wishes to thank both Ms. Lewis and Dr. Nardone for their help.

Published in 1999 by The Rosen Publishing Group, Inc.
29 East 21st Street, New York, NY 10010

First Edition
Copyright © 1999 by The Rosen Publishing Group, Inc.

Library of Congress Cataloging-in-Publication Data

Diamond, Shifra N.
    Everything you need to know about going to the gynecologist / Shifra Diamond.
        p. cm. — (The Need to know library)
    Includes bibliographical references and index.
    ISBN 0-8239-2839-X
    1. Teenage girls—medical examinations—Juvenile literature. 2. Gynecology—Juvenile literature. 3. Generative organs, Female—Diseases—Juvenile literature. 4. Obstetrics—Juvenile literature. 5. Sex instruction for youth—Juvenile literature. [1. Gynecology. 2. Sex instruction for girls.] I. Title. II. Series.
RG122.D53   1999
618.1dc21
                                         98–40929
                                            CIP
                                           AC

Contents

Introduction

If you are a teenager, chances are you have noticed changes in your body. Your figure may have become curvy. Your breasts have begun to develop and you've probably started wearing a bra. You may have started menstruating (getting your period).

Along with these physical changes come other new developments. Perhaps you have started noticing boys. Suddenly, dating and sex are on your agenda.

With these new issues come many new decisions. Some of these decisions, such as whether or when to have sex, and what kind of birth control to use, can change your life.

As you navigate these new choices, there are many people who can help. You might talk to a parent or friend. Or you might sort through feelings with a school counselor. When it comes to health issues, one person who can help is a gynecologist.

A gynecologist, or OB/GYN, is a doctor who has special training in women's sexual and reproductive health: breast care, menstrual health, and birth control.

You don't need to wait until you are sexually active before going to an OB/GYN. If you have painful periods, or other pain in your reproductive organs, a gynecologist can treat these problems. If you are thinking about having sex, a gynecologist can give you valuable information about birth control and preventing sexually transmitted disease (STDs).

Even if you are not sexually active, it's a good idea to get regular checkups from a gynecologist. This is part of becoming responsible for your own health and well-being, and becoming a woman.

But going to the gynecologist may seem scary or embarrassing, since the gynecologist looks at parts you usually keep covered. She may ask questions about sex, which you may still feel uncertain about. You probably also have many questions: Will you have to take off your clothes? What happens during the exam?

This book will tell you what to expect on your first visit to the gynecologist. It will talk about finding a gynecologist and describe what will happen once you get there. Going to a gynecologist doesn't have to be scary—when you know the facts.

Lastly, you will find resources for further information. Knowing these facts, you can make smart choices about your sexual and reproductive health.

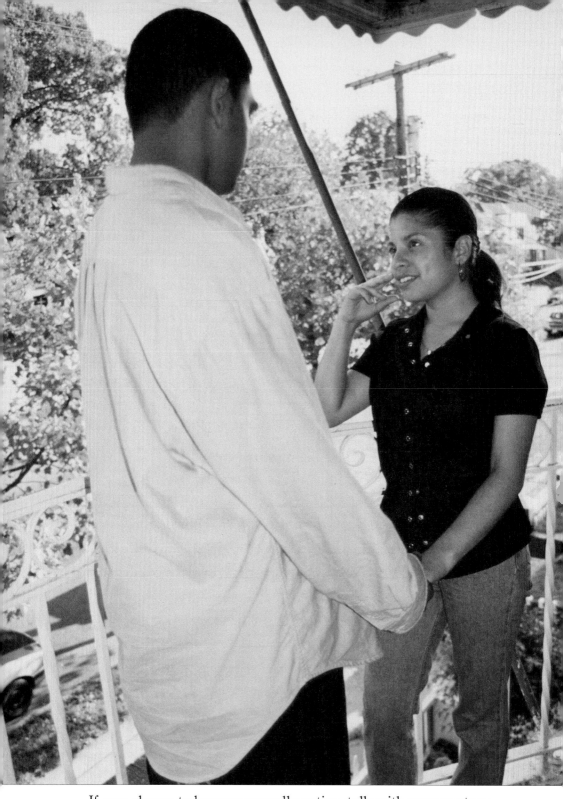

If you choose to become sexually active, talk with your partner and your gynecologist about being ready and being safe.

Chapter 1
Choosing a Gynecologist

*S*ari sits on her bed, nervously fiddling with the phone cord. In front of her is a telephone number for the local Planned Parenthood clinic. Every few minutes she picks up the receiver, dials two digits, and then hangs up.

Sari smiles when she realizes that this is what she used to do whenever she called Bobby. But now she and Bobby have been going out for two years. Recently, Sari and Bobby have been talking about having sex. Sari thinks she's ready. After all, she is seventeen. But she wants to be responsible. She will have sex only if she and Bobby use birth control. The problem was, she knew her mother would freak out if she asked her about it. So Sari talked to her school counselor. The counselor gave her the name of a clinic. At the clinic, she can get a checkup from a gynecologist and talk about her concerns about sex and birth control.

Sari remembers the counselor had said how proud she was of Sari for being so responsible. She smiles again. That made her feel good. She picks up the phone, and dials the full number. She'll make an appointment for Monday.

If you have recently learned that you need to see a gynecologist for the first time, you probably have many questions. Why is a gynecologist necessary? How should you go about finding one? Do you have to tell your mother? This chapter will give you some basic information about what you should know before scheduling your appointment.

What Is a Gynecologist?

A gynecologist is a doctor who takes care of women. He or she has special training in women's sexual and reproductive health: breast care, menstrual health, birth control and pregnancy, and sexually transmitted diseases.

Gynecologists are also trained in obstetrics, the care of pregnant women and childbirth. They are called obstetrician-gynecologists, or OB/GYNs. If you become pregnant, your OB/GYN can provide proper care so that you give birth to a healthy baby. In fact, an OB/GYN will probably be the one who delivers your baby.

Why Go to a Gynecologist?

Why not just go to a regular doctor? A gynecologist is a specialist. That means he or she has had extra training in gynecology. An OB/GYN is the best choice for assistance with health problems associated with menstruation and female reproductive organs.

Although you can still go to your family doctor for other health matters, gynecologist visits are an important part of growing up and taking care of yourself.

When Should You Start Going to a Gynecologist?

Traditionally, doctors have advised women to have their first gynecological checkup when they become sexually active or have reached the age of eighteen (whichever comes first). But if you are between the ages of thirteen and fifteen you may want to visit a gynecologist to talk about periods, birth control, and sexually transmitted diseases (STDs).

There are other reasons why you might need to see a gynecologist. If you are experiencing irregular or unusually heavy periods, if you are worried because you have never gotten your period, or if you think you may have a vaginal infection (which may not be sexually transmitted), it's a good idea to make an appointment, no matter what your age.

From then on, you should visit the gynecologist once a year.

Choosing a Gynecologist

In general, the best way to find a good doctor is by asking people you know for the names of their doctors.

When to See a Gynecologist

- When you start or are thinking of becoming sexually active (i.e., having intercourse)
- If you experience pain during your period or during sexual activity
- If you haven't gotten your period and are nearing age seventeen
- If you experience symptoms of STDs or other gynecological disorders
- When you are about eighteen, even if none of the above applies

This is called asking for a referral. Many teens use their mother's OB/GYN, or ask him or her to recommend someone. If you don't feel comfortable discussing this with your mother, ask a friend, a relative, your family doctor, or school nurse for referrals.

You can also call your local Planned Parenthood clinic. Many hospitals and women's organizations also have referral hotlines. Some hospitals also have clinics where you can pay on a sliding scale, depending on your income.

Something to remember: If your medical insurance is part of an HMO (health maintenance organization), you will probably have to use one of the doctors in its directory. For a list of doctors, call the customer service number at your HMO. Then ask friends and relatives if they're familiar with any of the doctors listed.

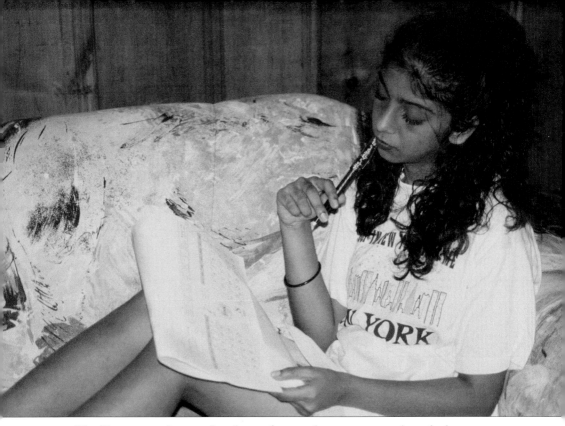

You'll want to know the date of your last menstrual period before you make an appointment with the gynecologist.

What Should You Look For in a Gynecologist?

When choosing a doctor, there are two qualities you should consider: First, make sure the doctor has been "board-certified" by the American Board of Obstetrics and Gynecology. This means that, after graduating from medical school and completing a four-year residency (special training course) in obstetrics and gynecology, the doctor has treated women's health conditions for at least two years and has passed an oral exam and a written test showing that he or she has the knowledge and skills to treat women.

It is also important that you feel comfortable with your

doctor. You may not know this until after your first appointment. But if you don't feel comfortable, don't hesitate to look for another doctor before your next checkup.

Choosing a Man or a Woman

In the past, most gynecologists, like most doctors, were men. But now, more and more women are becoming gynecologists.

Whether you choose a male or female doctor is up to you. Some women feel more comfortable with a female doctor. Other women do not care, or prefer to see a man. Whichever you choose, be assured that all gynecologists—both women and men—are trained to be very professional with their patients.

Do I Need to Tell My Mother?

Many teens worry about telling their mom, since even a routine gynecology checkup can raise sensitive issues about sexuality.

It's normal for teens to feel uncomfortable when talking about sex with their parents. But it is always a good idea to keep the lines of communication open. If that seems impossible in your situation, try to find a trusted adult you can talk to—an older friend, relative, guidance counselor, or clergy. Talking about it will give you the reassurance you need.

If you choose not to tell your mom, you can still make sure that your doctor visit is confidential. At Planned Parenthood clinics, for instance, you can get a complete gynecological checkup, as well as birth control, without a parent's permission.

Even a private doctor is required by law to keep your records confidential. That means that if you choose not to let your mother know what went on at your checkup, she'll never find out. But keep in mind that a diaphragm fitting or birth control pill prescription may turn up on a doctor's bill. So if your parents pay the bill (a likely scenario for most teens), talk to your gynecologist about what to do.

Making the Appointment

When you call the doctor's office to set up an appointment, the receptionist will need to know certain information: your name, age, address, phone number, type of medical insurance, and the reason for your visit. Don't hesitate to tell her if you want to get birth control or if you've been experiencing certain symptoms. Figure out in advance when you might be getting your period so that you can avoid scheduling an appointment at that time.

Of course, if you are experiencing painful symptoms, make an appointment as soon as possible.

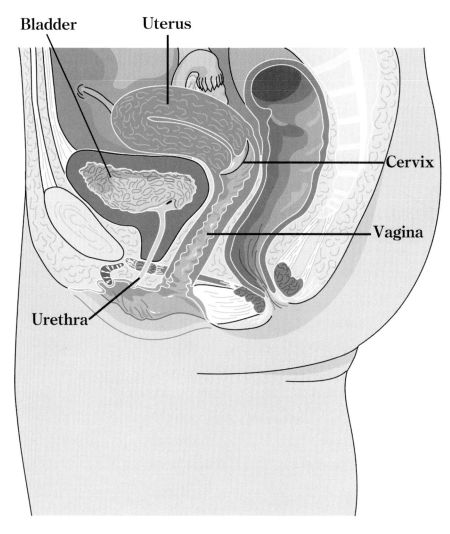

A cross-section of the female reproductive system.

Chapter 2

Getting to Know Your Body

At a gynecological exam, the doctor checks the health of your sexual and reproductive organs. But what exactly will the doctor see? Before your appointment, it's a good idea to get to know your own body. This chapter will answer some questions you may have: What do women's reproductive and sexual organs look like? How do they work together?

By becoming familiar with your sexual organs, you'll not only be ready for your appointment, but you can also make good choices about both your health and your sexual behavior.

Puberty: A Time of Changes

Puberty, which starts as you near your teens, is the time when your body gets ready for adult sexuality and child-bearing. During puberty, many changes occur in your body. Your breasts develop. Hair appears in your pubic area. Ovulation begins, and you begin to get your period (menstruate).

What sets these changes into motion? Puberty, and the entire reproductive cycle, is regulated by hormones, chemical messengers in the body. During puberty, your body starts producing more sex hormones. During your reproductive years, these hormones shift their balance each month. The shifts determine when you ovulate and when your period starts.

The Reproductive System

A woman's reproductive system is made up of many organs: the uterus, ovaries, and fallopian tubes; the vulva, clitoris, and vagina; and the breasts. Each plays a different part in reproduction.

The Vulva

A woman's outer genital area, called the vulva, is a soft, fleshy area covered with pubic hair.

Between the legs, the vulva is divided into two sets of labia (vaginal lips)—the outer lips (labia majora), and the inner lips (labia minora). Both are soft and sensitive to the touch. These lips partly cover three other areas of the vulva: the clitoris, the urethra (urinary opening), and the vagina.

The Clitoris

The clitoris (KLIT-o-riss) is the only organ in a

woman's body whose single purpose is sexual sensation. The tip (glans) of the clitoris is found toward the top of the vulva. It looks like a tiny knob covered by a hood. This is the most sensitive spot in the entire genital area, and when touched, can lead to an orgasm, a series of pleasurable sensations. The tip of the clitoris is connected to a network of muscles, veins, nerves, and tissue inside the pubic area that contribute to sexual arousal.

The Urethra

Right below the clitoris is the urinary opening. It looks like small dot or slit. This is the outer opening of the urethra, a short (about one and a half inches), thin tube that leads to the bladder.

The Vagina and Cervix

The vagina (or vaginal canal) is the opening to a woman's inner reproductive organs. When a woman has sexual intercourse, this is where the man's penis enters. During childbirth, a baby emerges. Inside the vagina are soft, sensitive folds of skin. The vaginal walls are lubricated with a natural fluid.

The innermost part of the vagina is called the cervix. The cervix is the base of the uterus (womb). It is a pliable, nose-shaped canal with a small dimple. The dimple is the opening into the uterus. When a woman gives birth, the cervix softens and expands enormously for the baby to come out.

The Uterus, Ovaries, and Fallopian Tubes

At the top of the vaginal canal, just below your bladder, are the reproductive organs: the uterus, ovaries, and fallopian tubes. These are the organs that work together to get an egg ready for conception.

The uterus, or womb, is a powerful muscle that holds the growing fetus when a woman is pregnant. When a woman is not pregnant, it is only about as big as a closed fist.

On either side of the uterus are the two ovaries. They are about the size and shape of unshelled almonds. The ovaries have two functions: they produce eggs (ova) and female sex hormones, including estrogen and progesterone.

At the top of the uterus, extending from both sides like ram's horns, are the two fallopian tubes. Sometimes called oviducts (literally, "egg tubes"), they are the tubes through which the egg travels each month from ovary to uterus. They are about four inches long. Inside are microscopic hairs (cilia) that propel the egg toward the uterus. The cilia are in constant motion. When sperm are inside, they also move the sperm toward the egg.

The Menstrual Cycle

The menstrual cycle (from the Latin word *mensis,* or "month") is the monthly cycle during which the reproductive organs prepare for the possibility of impregnation. When pregnancy doesn't happen, the body rids

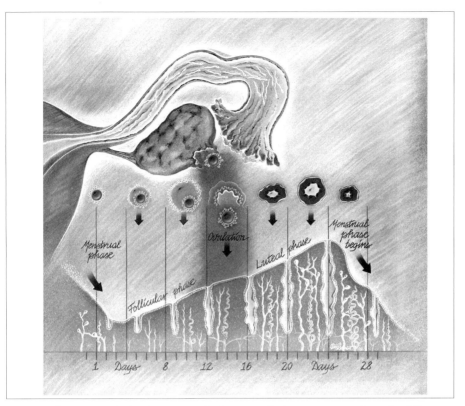

A diagram of the hormonal phases of the menstrual cycle. The lining of the uterus builds as an egg prepares to be released. Roughly fourteen days after that, if the egg is not fertilized, the lining is shed.

itself of the extra blood and nutrients that have gathered in the uterus to nourish the growing baby (fetus). This is the menstrual flow, or period. In most women the cycle takes about twenty-eight days.

Ovulation: The Egg's Journey Begins

Each month, in response to messages sent by hormones, one egg comes out of the ovary. This is called ovulation. (You probably won't notice ovulation, but you may feel a twinge or cramp in your lower stomach or back at this time.) After ovulation, the egg is swept into the funnel-

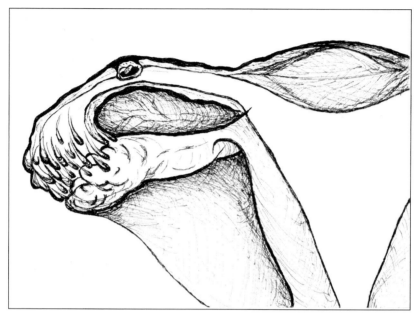

An egg travels through the fallopian tube on its way to the uterus.

shaped end of one of the fallopian tubes (oviducts) and begins its journey to the uterus, moved along by wave-like contractions of the tube.

If a man's sperm meets the egg while it is in the outer third of the fallopian tube (nearest the ovaries), the egg will be fertilized. Also called conception, this means a woman has become pregnant. It is most likely to occur within one day of ovulation, but it can happen anytime the egg is in the oviduct.

If the egg is fertilized, it will continue traveling toward the uterus, a process that takes five or six days. Then it will attach itself to the wall of the uterus and begin to grow and develop. In about nine months, a baby will be ready to be born.

If the egg is not fertilized, it flows out of the vagina during the menstrual period.

Menstruation

At the same time as the egg is making its way down the fallopian tube, the uterus is preparing for the embryo that might soon be developing. Its preparations are governed by hormones, especially estrogen and progesterone.

Just before ovulation, estrogen is released by the maturing egg. Estrogen increases the blood supply to the uterus and causes the uterine lining (endometrium) to grow and thicken in preparation for a potential embryo (a developing fetus). After the egg is released from the ovary, progesterone causes the endometrium to begin secreting substances to nourish the embryo. If the egg has been fertilized, it will begin to grow into an embryo once it reaches the uterus.

If the egg has not been fertilized, the ovary produces less and less estrogen and progesterone. As hormone levels drop, most of the uterine lining is shed. This is menstruation.

The bottom layer of the uterine lining remains to form a new lining. Then a new egg starts growing and secreting estrogen, a new uterine lining grows, and the cycle begins again.

Period Q & A

What is the normal age to get my first period?

Most girls start menstruating when they are twelve or thirteen. But starting any time from ages nine to sixteen is considered normal.

Can I menstruate without ovulating?

Yes, it is possible to get your period without having ovulated. This is called an annovulatory period. It is particularly common in young women, whose cycles are not yet regular.

How long does a period last?

Most women menstruate for four to six days. (The flow may stop and start). However, it is normal for a period to last from two to eight days. The whole monthly cycle is usually twenty to thirty-six days (twenty-eight days on average). Any cycle that is fairly regular is normal.

How much blood will I lose?

It may seem that you're bleeding a lot, but the usual discharge for a menstrual period is only about four to six tablespoons. Menstrual fluid also contains many substances besides blood (including the endometrium, or uterine lining). Although the amount of blood you lose is actually small, it can cause anemia, a lack of iron. For this reason, many women add iron supplements to their diets or eat iron-rich foods such as spinach, beans, or red meat.

Can anyone tell that I have my period?
People won't know unless you tell them.

Does it hurt?
Periods are often accompanied by cramps, but the actual flow shouldn't hurt. (See chapter 4 for information on cramps.)

Will I menstruate for the rest of my life?
Except for when you are pregnant, you should have a period every month until you reach your late forties or early fifties. Then menstruation and ovulation gradually stop, and a woman can no longer conceive a child. This is called menopause.

Chapter 3

The Gynecological Exam: What to Expect

*D*ear Emma,

I'm sorry I haven't written in a while. I've been really nervous about my first gynecologist visit. But I went today, and it was fine. The doctor was really nice. She listened to my questions and didn't lecture me when I told her I wanted birth control. The exam was a little embarrassing, but it was over pretty quickly. And now I have a diaphragm! (Of course, I'll still insist that Bobby use a condom.)

Anyway, just wanted to let you know that you have nothing to worry about when it's your turn to go to the gyn. I'll even go with you if you want. Talk to you soon!

Love, Sari

Like Sari, you too may be nervous about facing your first visit to the gynecologist. Will she ask you embarrassing questions? Will the examination hurt? Will you have to undress completely?

If the thought of getting a checkup makes you nervous, you are not alone. But chances are, like Sari, you'll find out it isn't as bad as you feared. This chapter will tell you what to expect at a regular gynecological checkup.

Before the Exam

Before starting the exam, the doctor will probably want to meet with you in her office or in the examining room to find out a bit about your background and your concerns. If you want to, you can ask your mom or a friend to come in with you for this discussion. But if you want to talk to the doctor about something confidential, ask your mom to wait outside.

You may want to write down any questions you have about your body or your health before your appointment. If you've scheduled your visit because of a specific problem, write down your symptoms, when they began, and whether they've gotten better or worse over time. If there is something you want to talk about, feel free to bring it up.

Don't worry if you forget to ask something, though. You can always call back after the appointment and talk to the doctor or a nurse over the phone.

Health History

One of the first things the doctor does is obtain a history of your health. You might be asked to fill out a form with this information. Once you have filled out the form, the doctor will talk to you about your answers.

The doctor may ask how old you were when you got your first period; the date your most recent period started, and whether it is regular; whether you are sexually active or are planning to be; whether you take birth control pills or other medications; and whether you are or ever have been pregnant. You will also be asked about any illnesses you've had and about your family health history.

It's a good idea to check with a parent or family member before your appointment to get this information. Or you could refer your gynecologist to your family doctor, who probably has this information in her files.

In addition to looking at your medical history, the doctor may ask about your health habits. If you smoke, use drugs or alcohol, or eat a high-fat diet, you should discuss this with your doctor. These habits not only have a bad effect on your overall health, but can increase your risk of certain gynecological disorders. Also, if you smoke or take drugs while you are pregnant, you can harm your baby.

One other piece of information you should take along is your insurance identification number and card, so that you can be billed properly. Be ready to give your card to the receptionist, either before or after your appointment.

Talking to Your Doctor: Honesty Counts

One thing your doctor will need to know is whether you are sexually active, at what age you began having sex, and other matters that you would not normally tell a stranger. You might feel squeamish about revealing these personal details. But remember, knowing about your sex life is part of a gynecologist's job. Without this information, the doctor would not be able to give you the best advice and care for your reproductive and sexual health. Your answers should be honest and open.

Don't worry, anything you tell your doctor will be kept confidential—no one else will know (not even your parents). In fact, doctors are required by law to keep your medical files confidential, unless it's about a life-threatening situation. Only by being honest will you be able to get the complete health care you need.

In the Examining Room

The physical exam has three parts: a check of your general health (weight, blood pressure, heartbeat), the breast exam, and the pelvic exam. After that, the doctor may perform some extra blood tests or cultures for sexually transmitted diseases or anemia (see page 25). The whole checkup usually takes no more than twenty minutes.

If this is your first time seeing a gynecologist, say so. Ask the doctor to go slowly and explain what she is doing. If at any time during the exam you feel uncomfortable, speak up.

Before the exam, the doctor may ask you for a urine sample, but even if she doesn't, it's a good idea to use the bathroom first, since a full bladder could interfere with the pelvic exam. Then, if you haven't done so already, it's time to change into the examining gown. (The opening usually goes in front.) Yes, you will need to remove all your clothes, including bra and underpants. But again, remember that seeing undressed women is just part of the doctor's job.

Breast Exam

The purpose of the breast exam is to make sure that your breasts are healthy. Because breast cancer is extremely rare in women younger than twenty-five, it is unlikely that any lump that is found would be cancer. However, there are some types of cysts (enlarged glands) and lumps (called fibroadenomas) found in young women that, though usually harmless, should be watched.

During the breast exam, the doctor will ask you to lie back on a table. She will look at your breasts to check their appearance. Then she will check for unusual lumps by touching your breasts. If your breasts are tender (common when breasts are growing and just before your period), it is usual to feel a bit of discomfort during this exam. But if anything hurts, don't be afraid to speak up.

Breast Self-Examination

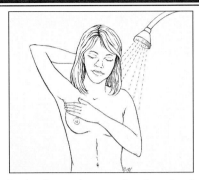

In the shower, keep one hand overhead and examine each beast with the opposite hand.

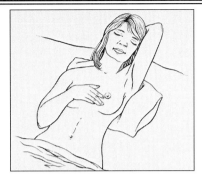

Lying in bed, place a pillow under one shoulder to elevate and flatten breast. Examine each breast with opposite hand, first with arm under head and again with arm at side.

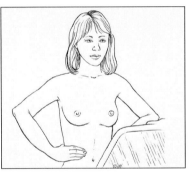

In front of a mirror, stand with hands resting on hips. Examine breasts for swelling, dimpling, bulges, and changes in skin.

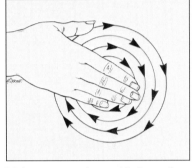

Make rotary motions–with flat pads, not tips of fingers–in concentric circles inward toward nipple. Feel for knobs, lumps, or indentations. Be sure to include the armpit area.

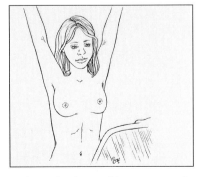

In front of mirror, with arms extended overhead, examine breasts for changes. This position highlights bulges and indentations that may indicate a lump.

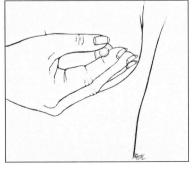

Squeeze nipples gently to inspect for any discharge. Report any suspicious findings to your doctor.

It's a good idea to do a breast self-exam at home every month. If you are not sure how to do this, ask the doctor or nurse to teach you.

The Pelvic Exam

After checking your breasts, the doctor does an exam of your pelvic organs. For this part of the exam, you will need to slide your feet into footrests (called stirrups) and lie on the table with your legs raised and knees spread apart. It's normal to feel uncomfortably exposed in this position. To put you at ease, the doctor may cover your lower body with a sheet. (Feel free to request a sheet if she doesn't offer one.)

As with the breast exam, the doctor will look first and then touch. First she looks at the outer genital area (vulva) and the opening to your vagina, making sure that everything looks fine. Then, to get a better view of the inside of the vagina and the cervix, she gently inserts a slender instrument called a speculum into the vagina.

The speculum is a tube-shaped instrument made of metal or plastic. Once inside, it opens slightly and holds the vaginal walls apart. (This shouldn't hurt, although you might feel some pressure. Try relaxing your muscles as much as possible and, if this doesn't help, tell the doctor. She can readjust the speculum or try a smaller size.)

The speculum lets the doctor see all the way in to your cervix. She will examine the walls of the vagina and check your cervix for anything unusual. Some doctors keep a hand mirror nearby and will let you look at your cervix.

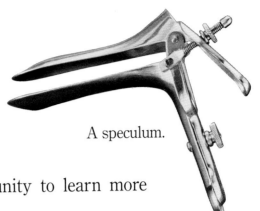

A speculum.

This is a good opportunity to learn more about your body.

During the short time the speculum is in place, the doctor also takes a sample of cells from the cervix to test for abnormal cell growth. This is called a Pap smear. She may also take a culture for gonorrhea and chlamydia, another culture to check for yeast infection or bacterial vaginisis, and a bit of vaginal discharge to examine for infection. This should not hurt, although you may have some spotting for a day or two after the test. (Spotting is more likely if you are pregnant or if you have a vaginal infection.) The cells are swabbed onto a slide and sent to a laboratory, where a trained technician will examine them. You should get a call from your doctor telling you the results within two weeks.

After the speculum is removed, the doctor will put on a clean plastic glove and insert one or two gloved fingers into the vagina. She will reach up to the cervix, while her other hand gently presses on your stomach from the outside. By doing this, she can feel the uterus, ovaries, and fallopian tubes. This test allows her to check their size, position, and shape. She can also locate any unusual growths, swelling, tenderness, or pain. You should feel some pressure, but not pain. If you do feel pain, let the doctor know.

Other Tests

Besides the Pap test and breast exam, there are a few other tests you can have done by an OB/GYN. Which ones you receive depends on your age and whether you are at risk for any disease. Tests for teens include:
- STD tests, including cultures for gonorrhea and chlamydia.
- HIV blood test to determine whether you have acquired the virus that can cause AIDS.
- Blood count, a test for detecting anemia (low iron) or other infection.
- Urinalysis, a test done on urine to look for changes that might be a sign of illness, especially urinary tract or bladder infection.
- Cholesterol test, a blood test done every five years to check levels of cholesterol, a substance that helps carry fat through the blood. If you have a high cholesterol count, your doctor may recommend a low-fat diet and other preventive health measures.
- Mammogram, an X ray of the breasts to detect breast cancer. This is generally done only when you are in your thirties or forties, but it may be done earlier if you have an unusual lump in your breast.

Methods of Birth Control

Going to the gynecologist is a good opportunity to find out about different kinds of birth control. Even if you're not yet sexually active, you can benefit from learning about birth control. That way, you'll have the facts when it's time to decide what's right for you.

Throughout this book, you've read about some methods of birth control, such as the condom or diaphragm. In this section you'll learn more about the pros and cons of those methods and others.

The Condom

The condom is a thin, flexible rubber sheath that fits over a man's penis. There is also a female condom, which fits inside a woman's vagina. A condom is the only form of birth control that is effective protection against sexually transmitted diseases.

You don't need a prescription from your doctor or gynecologist in order to get condoms; they're available at drugstores, supermarkets, and health clinics. Your gynecologist can help you learn how to use them properly.

The Birth Control Pill

Also known as "the Pill," birth control pills contain hormones that prevent pregnancy by holding back ovulation. Usually you have to take one pill a day, at the same time every day. Your period then comes during the last week of your packet of pills. Many teens take birth

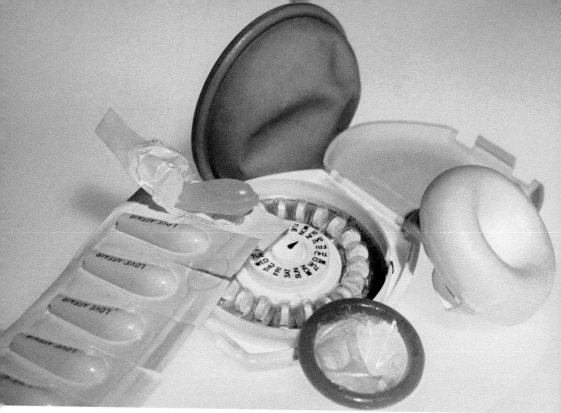

Contraceptives.

control pills not as birth control, but to regulate irregular periods.

Your gynecologist can prescribe birth control pills for you. But talk to him or her about possible side effects. Birth control pills offer no protection from sexually transmitted diseases, so they may or may not be right for you.

The Diaphragm and the Cervical Cap

Both of these methods of birth control are, together with the condom, known as barrier methods: they act as a barrier to prevent sperm from entering the uterus. The diapragm is a rubber, dome-shaped piece that fits snugly between the pubic bone and uterus, covering the cervix. The cervical cap is smaller and fits snugly over

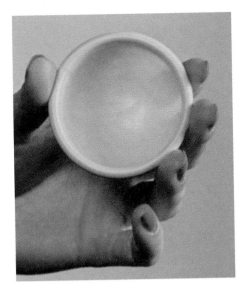

A diaphragm.

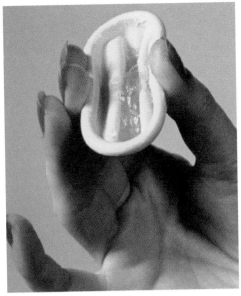

Contraceptive jelly in a diaphragm.

the cervix. Both can be inserted before having intercourse, together with a spermicide, and keep them in for up to eight hours after intercourse.

Your gynecologist can fit you for a diaphragm or cervical cap. But remember, neither of these methods is effective protection from sexually transmitted diseases.

Other Methods

You also may want to ask your gynecologist about other methods of birth control. Two of the most recent developments are hormone implants or injections made in your arm. They protect you from pregnancy, but not from sexually transmitted diseases.

You and your gynecologist may also need to weigh

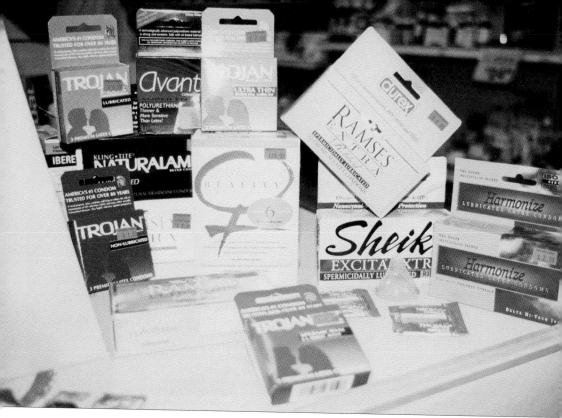

Condoms come in many varieties. In order to protect yourself from sexually transmitted diseases, use a condom together with a spermicide.

all your options before you try one of these methods. They're newer on the market, so the full range of their effects may not be known.

Myths (a.k.a. "Don't Try This!")

There are also many myths surrounding birth control. One is that there are certain times in your menstrual cycle when unprotected intercourse is safe. Another myth is that withdrawing the penis before ejaculation is effective birth control. No matter what your partner tells you, the truth is:

•It is unsafe to have unprotected intercourse, no matter what point you are in during your menstrual cycle.

•Withdrawing the penis before ejaculation is not safe, because sperm can enter the vagina before ejaculation.

If you ever have concerns about what is effective protection and what isn't, ask your gynecologist. No matter how strange your question may seem to you, chances are your doctor has heard (and answered) it before!

Your gynecologist can tell you more about the benefits and drawbacks of each method of birth control. Together you'll be able to decide on what works best for you.

Chapter 4

Reproductive Health: A Guide to Common Conditions

Chances are, your first gynecology checkup will be what doctors call a "well woman exam"—a routine checkup to confirm that you are healthy. But sometimes a missed period, serious cramps, or other symptoms can send you to the doctor.

What should you look for? When should you worry? How will the doctor treat the problem? In this chapter, you will learn about the most common health complaints associated with menstruation and women's reproductive organs—and what to do about them.

Menstrual Conditions

Amenorrhea: When Your Period Doesn't Show Up

What it is: There are two types of amenorrhea (the absence of menstrual periods): (1) If you have never gotten your period and you are nearing age seventeen (the latest age by which menstruation usually starts). (2) If you've gotten your period at least once, but since then it has stopped completely.

Why it happens: There are four common causes of consistently missed periods: (1) Pregnancy—if you have been having sexual intercourse. (2) Weight loss—due to eating disorders or heavy athletic training. (3) Hormone imbalance. (4) Stress. Severe anemia (low iron), as well as use of some prescription drugs and use of illegal drugs, can also make periods stop temporarily.

What to do: If you miss your period for more than two months (and you're not pregnant) or if you've never gotten a period, your gynecologist may prescribe progesterone pills (a type of hormone) to induce your period. If weight loss is the problem, returning to your minimum weight (i.e., when your body fat is one-quarter of your total weight) should make periods start again.

Premenstrual Syndrome (PMS)

What it is: PMS is the name for a group of physical and emotional changes that some women go through before their menstrual period begins. The symptoms follow a pattern: they reappear at about the same time each month and go away after your period has begun.

Symptoms: Physical changes: breast tenderness or swelling, bloating, weight gain, headache, fatigue, constipation, clumsiness. Emotional changes: depression,

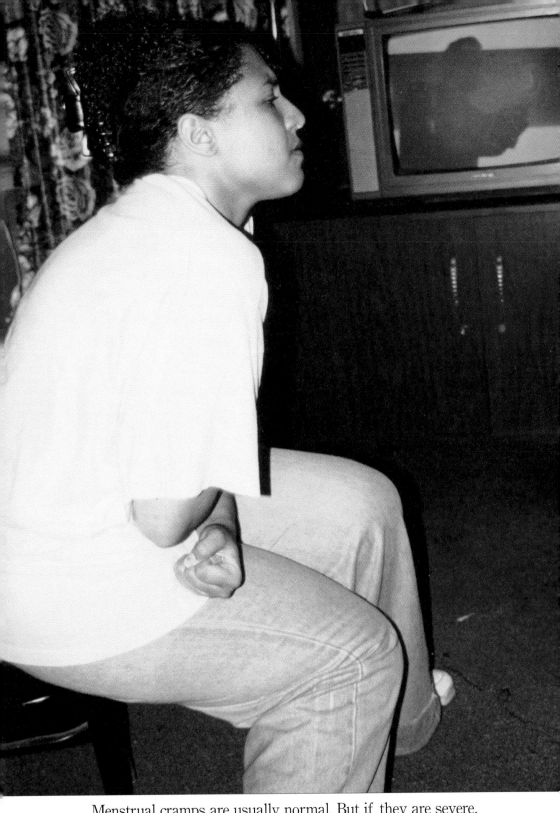

Menstrual cramps are usually normal. But if they are severe, talk to your gynecologist.

irritability, anxiety, tension, mood swings, inability to concentrate, change in sex drive. You don't need to have all of these to have PMS, and the severity of symptoms can vary from month to month.

Why it happens: So far, doctors do not know what causes PMS or why some women are affected more than others. Researchers are investigating whether estrogen and progesterone (the hormones that stimulate menstruation) may act with chemicals in the brain to cause some PMS symptoms.

What to do: There is no cure for PMS, but there are ways to cope. To prevent swelling, bloating or breast tenderness, steer clear of salt and caffeine for two weeks before your period. Reducing caffeine (found in coffee, tea, colas, and chocolate) can also calm anxiety, insomnia, and irritability. If you feel depressed, talk to a close friend, family member, or counselor. Schedule time for energizing exercise and make sure you get extra sleep.

Dysmenorrhea: The Very Painful Period

What it is: Menstrual cramps, sometimes accompanied by diarrhea, are the most common period complaint. But if they are exceedingly painful and are accompanied by other symptoms, such as nausea or vomiting, it may be a sign of a more serious condition.

Why it happens: Cramps occur when the uterus contracts to expel its endometrial lining. As the rhythmic contractions become longer and tighter they constrict;

this keeps oxygen from the muscles. This lack of oxygen is what we perceive as pain.

What to do: For normal cramps, try relaxation exercises, massage, and over-the-counter painkillers. Choose nonaspirin pain relievers containing ibuprofen. These can quickly offer relief by limiting the production of prostaglandins, the hormonelike substances that cause the uterus to contract. (By contrast, acetaminophen and acetaminophen-based pain relievers are not effective anti-prostaglandins, though they will reduce some discomfort.) If pain persists, see your gynecologist, who can prescribe stronger anti-prostaglandin medication and check for other physical causes. She may also prescribe birth control pills—by inhibiting ovulation and reducing menstrual flow, they also reduce cramps.

When Your Period Doesn't Go Away

What it is: Cycles that vary widely in length are common in teenagers. But if your cycle continues to be irregular more than a year after you begin menstruating, it's a good idea to get a checkup.

Why it happens: Usually this is due to changes in the balance of the hormones estrogen and progesterone. Bleeding for more than one week may also be caused by a uterine fibroid.

What to do: See your doctor. A thorough pelvic exam will determine if you have a fibroid. If not, birth control pills should put your cycle back on track.

When Your Period Is Unusually Heavy or Light

What it is: It is normal for menstrual flow to vary by day or month, especially in teenagers who are just beginning to menstruate. Bleeding or spotting between periods is also common and not usually cause for alarm. But prolonged, heavy, or irregular bleeding can also indicate more serious conditions, so see your doctor.

Why it happens: If you do not ovulate regularly (common in teens whose cycles are just getting established), your body can experience a buildup of estrogen, which leads to late periods and very heavy bleeding. Other causes of abnormally heavy periods include pregnancy or miscarriage, STDs, cervical problems, or vaginitis. Taking amphetamines or over-the-counter diet aids can also increase menstrual flow and cramping.

What to do: If you have light, irregular bleeding, your doctor may suggest waiting a month or two to see if your system rights itself. You may be able to stabilize your menstrual flow by reducing stress and changing your diet. For heavy bleeding, she might prescribe estrogen pills. And ask your doctor about iron pills to offset anemia (low iron) from blood loss.

Conditions of Uterus and Ovaries
Endometriosis

What it is: Endometriosis is a chronic condition in which tissue that looks and acts like the inner lining (endometrium) of the uterus grows outside of the uterus. It may be attached to the ovaries, the intestines, or another part of the lower abdomen, but it is affected by female hormones as if it were in the uterus. At the end of each month, the tissue bleeds, but since the fluid cannot be flushed freely out of the body, it builds up inside, making nearby tissue swollen and painful. Often endometriosis causes pain that begins several days before the beginning of menstrual bleeding and is sometimes accompanied by spotting (slight bleeding).

Symptoms: Some women with endometriosis have no symptoms. For others, though, it can be extremely painful, especially during menstruation, ovulation, and/or sexual activity. It can cause pain in the pelvic area and lower back, extremely heavy menstrual flow, fatigue, and intestinal upset during your period.

Why it happens: No one knows exactly what causes endometriosis, although it may be genetic. Some doctors think it occurs when menstrual tissue backs up through the fallopian tubes, implants itself in the abdomen, and grows.

Who is at risk: Any woman can get endometriosis. Although people once thought only women in their late twenties or thirties were at risk, we now know that many women experience the first symptoms before age twenty-five.

How to find out if you have it: If you have symptoms of endometriosis, see your doctor. She may be able to diagnose it by placing her hand on your stomach during the pelvic exam. Sometimes, though, an ultrasound test or laparoscopy is needed. During laparoscopy, a light attached to a tube is inserted into a tiny cut in the abdomen so that the surgeon can see endometrial implants.

What to do about it: The most common treatment is to take hormone pills, which stop the ovary from producing estrogen (and also stop menstruation). Sometimes doctors prescribe oral contraceptives, which also regulate the period. In more serious cases, you may need to have surgery to remove the growth. Without treatment, endometriosis can lead to serious health problems, such as infertility, ruptured ovarian cysts, and problems with pregnancy.

It's a good idea to find a support group, such as the Endometriosis Association, to get information and share with others who understand what you are going through.

Pelvic Inflammatory Disease (PID)

What it is: Infection of the lining of the uterus, the fallopian tubes, and/or ovaries. It is caused primarily by sexually transmitted diseases (STDs) that spread to these organs. Nearly 1 million women in the United States are reported to develop PID each year, and about 300,000 women are hospitalized. Yet many cases of PID are undiagnosed. PID is an extremely serious problem that needs prompt and skilled attention.

Symptoms: The most common symptom is pain—tightness or pressure in the reproductive organs or an occasional dull ache in the lower abdomen. It may be mild or strong. It may be located in the middle or on one or both sides of your lower abdomen.

There are many other symptoms that can appear, depending on what is causing the infection, how long you've had it, and which organ is infected: pain or bleeding during or after intercourse; irregular bleeding or spotting; abnormal or bad-smelling discharge from the vagina or urethra; increased menstrual cramps; increased pain during ovulation; frequent urinating, burning, or inability to empty bladder; swollen abdomen; chills; swollen lymph nodes; sudden high fever or a low-grade fever that can come and go; lack of appetite, nausea, or vomiting; pain around the kidneys or liver; lower back or leg pain; feelings of weakness, tiredness, or depression; diminished sex drive.

Why it happens: Most cases of PID (90 to 95 percent) are caused by the microorganisms responsible for STDs, such as gonorrhea and chlamydia, which enter the body during sexual contact with an infected person. (Although men have few symptoms of PID, they can carry organisms that cause it, so your partner should be tested and treated as well, and should always use a condom.)

Who is at risk: Anyone can get PID, but women are at higher risk for developing PID if they have unprotected sexual intercourse.

Complications: If untreated, PID can cause chronic pain and can lead to serious health complications, spreading to the liver or bowels and causing infertility or peritonitis, an inflammation of the abdomen which can be a life-threatening condition. In the most extreme cases, untreated PID can result in death.

How to prevent PID: To prevent PID, you need to prevent STDs. Always use a condom during sex, especially if either of you has more than one sexual partner.

Uterine Fibroids

What they are: Uterine fibroids are solid, harmless (benign) tumors (growths of cells that serve no biological purpose). They appear in the lining or muscle of the uterus, or along its exterior, and can often change its size and shape.

Symptoms: Small fibroids usually cause no symptoms. If you have many fibroids, or if they are very large, you might experience pain or very heavy menstrual flow. Depending on where they are located and how big they are, fibroids can also cause urinary problems or pain in the stomach or back.

How to diagnose it: Fibroids can be diagnosed during a routine pelvic exam. Because fibroids keep growing, ask your doctor how many you have and how big they are. If they have grown no further when you have a second exam six months later, you'll just need a yearly checkup.

Who is at risk: About 30 percent of all women develop fibroids by the time they are thirty-five.

Why it happens: It is not known exactly what causes fibroids, but doctors believe that their growth is related to the body's production of estrogen. They tend to grow more quickly if you are pregnant.

What to do: Yoga exercises may ease feelings of heaviness and pressure. In many cases no treatment is necessary, but if you have excessive bleeding, pain, urinary difficulties, or problems with pregnancy, you may want to have the fibroids removed.

Ovarian Cysts

What they are: A simple ovarian cyst is an abnormal, fluid-filled sac that develops when a follicle in the ovary fails to rupture and release an egg. Cysts usually disappear by themselves, though sometimes they have to be removed.

Symptoms: Ovarian cysts are relatively common and often don't cause any discomfort. But you might experience pain during intercourse, irregularities in your normal menstrual cycle, an unfamiliar pain or discomfort in your lower abdomen at any point during the cycle, and unexplained abdominal swelling.

Why it happens: If you frequently get cysts, it may indicate a hormone imbalance, which can be caused by stress and may disappear if you change your diet or reduce stress.

What to do: Most ovarian cysts disappear on their own. If you have an ovarian cyst—which your doctor can diagnose during a pelvic exam—she may suggest you wait a few months to see if it goes away. If it persists, a doctor may use ultrasound to see if it is harmful and

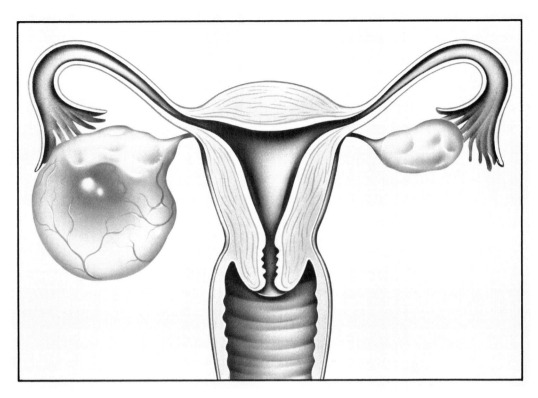

An ovarian cyst may go away on its own; however, if pain persists, you may want to have it removed.

should be removed. She also may prescribe birth control pills to regulate your hormones.

Conditions of the Vagina and Urinary Tract
Urinary Tract and Bladder Infections

What it is: UTIs, which are very common, are an infection of the urinary tract. The infection can happen in the urethra or the bladder. (More seriously, infection occasionally spreads to the kidneys.) About one in five women will have at least one urinary tract infection at some point in her life. Many women have more than one. Fortunately, most UTIs are not serious. They are easily treatable with antibiotics.

Symptoms: The first sign is a sudden strong urge to urinate every few minutes, followed by a sharp pain or burning sensation in the urethra, even though almost no urine comes out. This cycle repeats several times a day or night. You may also have pain or soreness in the lower abdomen, back, or sides.

Why it happens: UTIS are usually caused by bacteria, which travel from the bowel to the urethra and bladder (and occasionally to the kidneys). Women can also get urinary tract infections after sexual intercourse, when bacteria from the vaginal area can be brought into the urethra. STDS, such as trichomoniasis and chlamydia, can also cause UTIS.

What to do: See your doctor—especially if symptoms continue for forty-eight hours, or go away and come back. Call the doctor right away if you also have chills, fever, vomiting, or pain in the kidneys (which may mean the infection has spread to the kidneys, a serious problem that requires immediate medical treatment), if there is blood or pus in your urine, if you are pregnant, have diabetes, or had kidney or urinary tract infections when you were a child.

The doctor will give you a urine test and a pelvic exam to rule out other infections. If you have a UTI, she'll probably prescribe antibiotics, which you should take for seven to ten days. (Be sure to take all the medicine even if symptoms disappear more quickly, or the infection may come back.) About a week after treatment, you'll have a follow-up urine test to be certain the

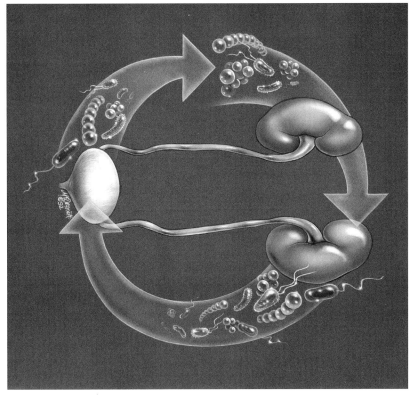

If a urinary tract infection is untreated, bacteria may spread to the bladder and kidneys.

infection is cured. If your UTI comes back frequently (for instance, every other week), your doctor may prescribe a low dose of antibiotic to be taken each day or every time you have sex.

Vaginal Infections (Vaginitis)

What it is: An infection of the vaginal walls and vulva.

Symptoms: Yellowish or bad-smelling vaginal discharge, mild or severe itching and burning of the vulva, chafing of the thighs, and occasionally frequent urination.

Why it happens: Vaginal infections happen when yeast or fungi in the vagina multiply and release waste that, in large amounts, irritates the vaginal walls. Infections

How to Prevent Urinary Tract and Vaginal Infections

•Practice good personal hygiene. Each day, gently wash the skin around the rectum and vagina. Before and after intercourse, wash again. Use nonsoap cleansers for sensitive skin.

•After going to the bathroom, always wipe from front to back (so bacteria from the bowels don't enter the vagina or urethra).

•Make sure your sexual partners are clean. Always use a condom during sexual intercourse, and don't have intercourse when you or your partner have any kind of infection.

•For lubrication during sex, use a sterile, water-soluble jelly (such as KY jelly or spermicidal jelly).

•During sexual intercourse, try positions that cause less friction to the urethra. If you experience pain during sexual intercourse, ask your partner to stop.

•Don't douche, unless your doctor has specifically recommended it.

•If you often get vaginal infections, avoid using the diaphragm and tampons.

•Cut down on coffee, alcohol, sugar, and carbohydrates: Diets high in sugar can change the normal chemical balance of the vagina.

•Drink plenty of fluids to flush bacteria out of your urinary system.

•Eat lots of vitamin C. It makes the urine acidic, which helps keep potentially harmful bacteria in check.

•Empty your bladder completely as soon as you need to (or every 2-3 hours). Urinate right after sex to flush out bacteria that entered the urethra during intercourse.

•Wear cotton underwear. Cotton "breathes," and doesn't trap moisture like ther fabrics.

•Take care of yourself. Not getting proper rest or nutrition makes you more susceptible to infection.

can also occur when the vagina's pH balance changes (due to douching, taking birth control pills or antibiotics) and can be caused by cuts and irritation in the vagina (from using tampons, having intercourse without enough lubrication, or inserting an object into the vagina). You can catch an infection from a partner. If you are stressed out or not getting enough sleep or eating right, you might also be more likely to get a vaginal infection.

What to do: See your doctor. She will prescribe an antibiotic cream or pill, which kills infection-causing bacteria.

Pain During Intercourse

What it is: Pain during sexual intercourse (called dyspareunia) is fairly common and should not be cause for embarrassment.

Symptoms: There are three main types of pain during intercourse: lack of lubrication in the vagina, vaginal muscle spasm (vaginismus)—both of which can occur at the opening of the vagina or within its walls—and pain deep inside, which happens when the penis touches the back of the vagina. All of these can range from very mild, occasional discomfort to severe pain that makes intercourse impossible.

Why it happens: Both physical causes and emotional issues can contribute to pain. Often these work together. Soreness and dryness in the outer half of the vagina can result from infections, such as vaginitis, bladder or urinary tract infections, or STDs such as herpes or trichomoniasis. Pain deep inside the vagina is usually a warning sign of ovarian cysts, infection of the uterus or fallopian tubes, or endometriosis.

Sometimes, after a woman has had painful intercourse for any of these reasons, the fear of pain will start to reduce her normal lubrication or tighten the muscles at the opening of her vagina. This muscle spasm, called vaginismus, is itself painful and sometimes can prevent entry of the penis. Vaginismus can also result from purely emotional reactions, especially tension, discomfort with the relationship or with the prospect of having sex, or memories of past sexual traumas, such as rape or sexual abuse.

Myths about painful intercourse: Women often think that pain happens because their vagina is too small, or because their partner is "too large." Neither is usually true.

A woman's vagina can expand to permit the birth of a baby. Studies show that an erect penis is about the same size in all men, no matter what the size before erection.

What to do about it: A thorough pelvic exam by your gynecologist should determine if you have an infection or other condition. You also might try relaxation exercises. If you think your problem might stem from discomfort with your relationship or other emotional issues, talking to a counselor may help.

A Final Word

Now that you know the facts, going to the gynecologist may seem a lot easier than you thought. Remember, going to the gynecologist is one way to become responsible for your own health and well-being. It's part of becoming a woman.

It's a good idea to keep learning as much as you can, even after that first appointment is over. At the end of this book you can find many resources where you can find more information. These organizations and others will help you make healthy choices throughout your life.

Glossary

amenorrhea Absence of menstrual period.

birth control pill A pill taken to regularize periods and prevent pregnancy.

breast The part of a woman's body containing a mammary gland.

cervical cap A barrier method of birth control worn over the cervix.

cervix The opening to the uterus.

clitoris The organ in a woman's body that gives sexual pleasure.

condom A sheath worn on the penis during intercourse to prevent pregnancy.

contraceptive Any device that prevents pregnancy.

diaphragm A barrier method of contraception; a flexible rubber dome that fits over the cervix.

dysmenorrhea The syndrome of having painful menstrual periods.

endometriosis A condition in which the tissue like lining of the uterus grows outside the uterus.

fallopian tube The tube connecting an ovary to the uterus.

gynecologist A doctor who specializes in women's reproductive health.

HMO Health Maintenance Organization; an organization that provides medical insurance.

mammogram A test on the breast to detect cancer.

menstruation The shedding of the uterine lining, occurring in women approximately every 28 days.

OB/GYN An obstetrician/gynecologist, a doctor who specializes in women's reproductive health.

obstetrics The care of pregnant women.

ovarian cyst A fluid-filled sac that develops when a follicle in the ovary fails to rupture and release an egg.

ovary The gland that produces the female sex hormones estrogen and progesterone.

oviduct The funnel-shaped end of a fallpian tube.

ovulation The release of an egg by the ovary.

Pap test A test run on cells taken from the cervix, checking for abnormalities.

pelvic inflammatory disease Infection of a woman's internal reproductive organs.

pregnancy Carrying a developing fetus within the body.

premenstrual syndrome A set of physical and emotional symptoms, such as bloating and irritability, that occur in a woman prior to the menstrual period.

sexually transmitted disease A disease spread through sexual intercourse.

speculum A tube-shaped instrument that holds the vaginal walls open during a gynecological exam.

urinary tract infection A bacterial infection causing inflammation of the urethra, kidneys, and bladder.

uterine fibroid A benign tumor that grows inside or outside the uterus.

uterus The muscle inside of which a fetus grows.

vagina The opening to a woman's inner reproductive organs.

vaginitis An infection of the vaginal walls and vulva

vulva A woman's outer genital area.

Where to Go for Help

Health Information
American College of Obstetricians and Gynecologists (ACOG)
409 West 12th Street, SW
Washington, DC 20024-2188

Endometriosis Association
8585 North 76th Place
Milwaukee, WI 53223
In the United States: (800) 992-3636
In Canada: (800) 426-2363

Women's Health Information Center
P.O. Box 192
West Somerville, MA 02144

http://www.gurl.com
An on-line magazine for girls that deals with issues such as body image, self-esteem, and sexuality.

Sexually Transmitted Diseases
AIDS for Teens Hotline
(800) 234-8336

CDC National STD Hotline
(800) 227-8922
CDC National AIDS Hotline
(800) 342-AIDS
(800) 344-SIDA (en español)

Safer Sex Page
Web site: http://www.safersex.org/

Pregnancy and Contraception

Planned Parenthood, Inc.
26 Bleecker Street
New York, NY 10003
(212) 274-7200
(800) 829-7732
Offers birth control services, pregnancy tests, prenatal care, STD education and treatment, AIDS testing, and HIV counseling.

Support for Gays, Lesbians, and Bisexuals

The Gay and Lesbian National Hotline
(888) 843-4564

Advice and Counseling

Covenant House Nineline
(800) 999-9999
Crisis intervention for all teenagers, particularly runaways and homeless youth.

The National Eating Disorders Organization (NEDO)

62655 South Yale Street
Tulsa, OK 74136
(918) 481-4044

Rape, Abuse, Incest National Network (RAINN)

(800) 656-HOPE
For victims of any kind of sexual assault; call this number to be automatically connected to a crisis center in your area.

Safe Choice Hotline

(800) 878-2437
Counseling and information for teens, especially about pregnancy and STD prevention.

In Canada

Hassle Free Clinics/AIDS Committee
556 Church Street, #2
Toronto, ON M4Y 2E3
(416) 922-0603

For Further Reading

Bell, Ruth. *Changing Bodies, Changing Lives: A Book for Teens on Sex and Relationships.* New York: Vintage Books, 1988.

Boston Women's Health Book Collective. *The New Our Bodies, Ourselves.* New York: Touchstone, 1992.

Moe, Barbara. *Everything You Need to Know About Sexual Abstinence.* New York: Rosen Publishing Group, 1996.

——. *Sex Ed: Growing Up, Relationships, and Sex.* New York: Dorling Kindersely Limited, 1997.

Shire, Amy. *Everything You Need to Know About Being HIV-Positive.* New York: Rosen Publishing Group, 1996.

Stoppard, Dr. Miriam. *The Breast Book.* New York: Dorling Kindersley Limited, 1996.

White, Evelyn C., ed. *The Black Women's Health Book: Speaking for Ourselves.* Seattle: Seal Press, 1990.

Woods, Samuel G. *Everything You Need to Know About STD: Sexually Transmitted Disease.* New York: Rosen Publishing Group, 1997.

Index

About the Author
Shifra N. Diamond is a freelance writer, editor, and educator living in New York City. She has written about women's health for *Mademoiselle, Brides,* and teaches gender studies at The New School. She holds a master's degree in English literature from Washington University.

Photo Credits
Cover, pp. 8, 13, 38, 42 by Les Mills; p. 2 by Ira Fox, pp. 21, 22, 31, 33, 36, 37, 51, 53 by © Custom Medical Stock Photo.